WALL PILATES
WORKOUT
FOR
BEGINNERS

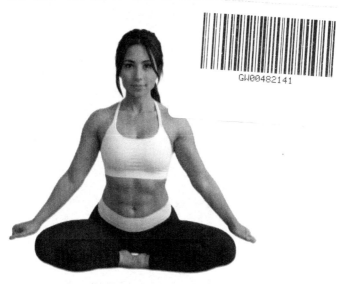

**Stretch and Strengthen Your Way
to a Stronger Core Using Pilates
on Any Blank Wall**

RICHARD L. LYONS

This book is a work of nonfiction. The information and opinions expressed in this book are those of the author and do not necessarily reflect the views of the publisher.

GAIN ACCESS TO MORE BOOKS FROM ME

TABLE OF CONTENT

INTRODUCTION

Elle stepped on the scale once again hoping for a lower number, but sighed seeing she still weighed 178 pounds - same as last week and the week before. Though only 27 years old, Elle felt her metabolism slowing down more each year. She looked at the tight pencil skirt in her closet and frowned, lacking motivation to keep trying to zip it up.

Sitting at her cramped New York apartment that night eating takeout and mindlessly scrolling social media, one post caught Elle's eye - a before and after transformation using something called "Wall Pilates." Intrigued, Elle clicked and read an excerpt from a new book called "Wall Pilates Workout for Beginners." The next day she ordered it on Amazon expecting quick results like the other failed fitness trends she had tried.

The book arrived and Elle eagerly read through the introduction learning how Wall

Pilates builds core muscles that support the spine and improve posture. The essential techniques looked simple enough - presses, planks, stretches using her blank living room wall. Elle followed the clear instructions starting with 30 minute beginner routines. After just 2 weeks Elle noticed her stomach and sides were surprisingly more toned. By a month in, she squeezed into her goal skirt with an inch to spare!

Now 6 months since starting Wall Pilates, Elle maintains her 30 pound weight loss easily. She feels stronger than her college cheerleading days. Best of all Elle gained confidence in herself again rather than just her appearance. She stands taller, works out consistency, and explores new hobbies besides the usual happy hours with friends. Wall Pilates gave Elle the jumpstart toward her healthiest and happiest self yet.

***

Pilates has become one of the most popular and proven workouts for building whole body strength, balance, and flexibility. For decades, enthusiasts have praised what Joseph Pilates originated nearly a century ago - a system that uniquely transforms bodies with dramatic results, using just simple and strategic mat exercises. What started as "Contrology", a set of 34 moves for injured WWI soldiers, is now a worldwide cultural fitness phenomenon, and for good reason. The benefits of a regular Pilates practice are vast, helping practitioners lose weight, recover faster, increase stamina, and gain mobility with less strain or chance of reinjury. Pilates advances bodies of all types to levels they never imagined - a testament to the universal genius of Joseph Pilates and his timeless, adaptable method.

While mat Pilates provides an effective strengthening option to those with space limitations, the wall offers yet a new dimension of resistance, stability, and alignment guidance. Free and requiring no equipment, wall workouts allow gravity and body leverage to put muscles through challenging new planes of motion. The blank canvas of any vertical surface combined with Pilates principles doubles the exercise possibilities, without the strain or limitations of reformers or gym machines. Wall Pilates unlocks full ranges by using the core to control springy movements rather than rigid presses. The bounce back effect hones power and balance dynamically by keeping tension fluid yet precisely muscle focused.

From tight city apartments like this author's own New York flat to remote islands or desert camps, the only equipment one ever needs is the arm's reach of an unobstructed wall. This makes Wall Pilates the perfect portable practice requiring just shoes or bare feet and workout wear with stretch. Complete core fitness can happen anytime with minimal space but maximum effectiveness. Consider this your guide to exploring Pilates in a whole new direction.

A Brief History of Pilates

Born in Germany in 1880, Joseph Pilates suffered from a weak and sickly youth plagued by rickets, asthma, and rheumatic fever that continued into his late teens. Inspired by Greek and Roman exercise regimens, Pilates developed a unique conditioning routine called "Contrology" to strengthen his underdeveloped body. Mixing Eastern and Western techniques like yoga, tai chi, and ancient Roman fitness traditions, Pilates emphasized full controlled movements, posture alignment, flexibility/balance training, and breath-centered energy. He believed mental and spiritual health were just as crucial as physical, an integrated mind-body approach.

After successfully transforming himself into a champion diver, boxer and gymnast, Pilates then worked with WWI internees detained at camp. There he refined 34 floor-based mat movements using springs or straps that adapted exercises to rehabilitate bedridden and wheelchair patients. Word spread of miraculous injury recoveries, drawing police and army recruits to attend his classes in the late 1920's back in Germany Despite warnings, the outspoken Pilates rejected rising Nazi propaganda and soon fled Germany to England for the decade. While there, famed Scotland Yard detectives and Royal National Ballet dancers alike raved of increased stamina and strength plus faster healing gained under his tutelage.

In 1926, Pilates sailed with his wife to New York on the HMS Queen Mary in hopes of reaching a wider audience very receptive at the time to health and body consciousness trends. After initially training some of New

York's elite, he opened his and his wife's signature "Pilates Studios of Fifth Avenue" in 1939. Over the next forty years until his death in 1967, their Manhattan studio trained A-list Hollywood celebrities like Martha Graham along with prominent athletes, politicians, CEOs and socialites. Around 1945, Pilates designed the first spring-based Reformer equipment to offer varied resistance and joint mobility. He later created the "Wunda Chair", "Cadillac", and "Ladder Barrel" to expand his no-impact training devices.

Such revolutionary gear also allowed Pilates methods to be taught after his passing in other studios worldwide. Dancers, fitness pros, physical therapists and more spread his teachings so comprehensively that Pilates forms the core (pun intended) of conditioning programs today from sports training to senior activities to physical rehabilitation. In the last two decades, Pilates earned mainstream recognition as a premier way for anybody to realign posture, develop strong flexible muscles, heal quicker with less pain, and integrate mind-body awareness for greater wellness benefits.

Why Wall Pilates Maximizes Core Results

As Joseph Pilates said, "Physical fitness is the first requisite of happiness." The core always serves as the source of all movement, balance, stability and strength that allows bodies to excel and feel empowered in motion. Pilates so effectively strengthens the inner powerhouse from pelvis to solar plexus with functional exercises that activate multiple muscles simultaneously in a safe joint-friendly manner. Core muscles groups challenge balance while aligning essential areas like shoulders and spine. Total body fitness emerges from a toned solid center that improves daily life performance and confidence. Jerome started on his living room carpet realizing the floor limited core engagement that midair suspension against gravity amplifies. He found vertical planes intensified the resistance by forcing core muscles to resist extension of legs and arms pulled by gravity away from centers. Wall space brought springy elasticity for abs to reinforce while limbs freely stretch in all planes. Whether upright or supine, vertical surface area provides the core unique multidimensional challenges to stabilize postures impossible on just flat floors.

With hundreds more options, wall space allows users to progress from beginner to advanced levels gradually unlike limited mat routines that lose effectiveness over time and joint safety. Workouts turn more functional, adaptive and progressive using personalized friction, spring and gravity factors. Wall space also aligns format perfectly to target trouble areas like tight shoulders or hips with adjustable decompression stretches. Open chests counteract rounded shoulders while tight quads and hip flexors that prevent twisting are elongated. Most importantly, wall traction bolsters spinal flexibility and joint mobility safely to reduce or eliminate chronic pain. By centering workouts around versatile wall space, Pilates soars to new heights strengthening cores beyond expectations.

Essential Wall Pilates Gear

The beauty of Wall Pilates lies in simple basics required that use no bulky equipment taking up space. Ultimately just core bodyweight and reliable walls provide all one needs to facilitate upper thresholds of strength gains, flexibility increases, stability improvements and postural realignments. Essentially the only Wall Pilates workout necessities include:

- Athletic shoes for grip and support or bare feet to gauge balance. Thick socks also aid sliding motions on carpets.

- Fitted pants and tops to prevent tangling but not restrict. Stretch fabrics like cotton blends, sweat wicking performance wear, leggings/tights or athletic shorts work well.

- A solid blank vertical surface area at least 6 feet wide by 8 feet tall. Use empty living room/bedroom walls, building exteriors, hallways, decks, garages or outdoor shed/barn walls weather permitting. Travel bands also convert hotel rooms instantly.

- Exercise/Yoga Mats enhance padding, traction and barrier from cold hard surfaces. Plus eases sliding seated movements like heel slides or mudras.

- Resistance Bands/Mini-Bands boost lower/upper body toning, mimic

Pilates rings, and increase cardio burn with rhythmic pulsing motions.

That's it! Simply body, breath and bare wall space启动all one needs to strengthen like never before. While Pilates reformers or balls bring value, walls transform abilities exponentially without recurring fees or reliance on machines as Joseph Pilates intended. Now let's explore how to maximize wall workouts for fast flexible results!

How to Use This Wall Pilates Beginners Guide

This definitive guide unlocks Wall Pilates full potential with progressive step-by-step techniques for all skill levels. While seemingly basic moves facilitate dramatic strength and flexibility shifts from core to limbs. Strategies suit any schedule or space while preventing strain or repetition related injuries common in conventional training. With clear visual demonstrations and accompanying tips, Wall

Pilates empowers all ages and body types for lifelong wellness.

Chapter 1 covers core concepts and beginner flows to establish solid foundations in proper breathing, form, spinal alignment and core rooting. Without strong bases in technique and posture, progress stalls and strain emerges. Core control always takes priority over range or depth movements in Wall Pilates.

Chapter 2 guides breathing focused mobility warm ups using myofascial release, gentle contractions and traction. Stretching increases joint circulation and elongates muscles before workouts, preventing torn tissues or imbalances long term. Proper warmup preps the body optimally for any activity in just minutes.

Chapters 3-6 provide Wall Pilates exercise progressions by body area - upper body/arms, core/abs, lower body/glutes/thighs with a flexibility cooldown chapter. Step-by-step instructions demonstrate proper pacing, positioning, adjustment tips and difficulty levels from basic to advanced. Cues direct focus to working muscle groups with holistic whole body awareness. Simply progress or regress moves by adjusting angles and range of motion based on individual ability. Rest days in between sessions advised.

The Conclusion covers how to effectively sequence daily, weekly and monthly Wall Pilates routines for balanced strength building across opposing muscles and sides. Holistic symmetry prevents fitness plateaus and overuse related strains. Sample beginner and intermediate flows provided along with space to design your own custom programs. Lastly discover lifestyle integration bonuses from nutrition to sleep hygiene.

Transform more than just your body but your entire mindset toward lifelong wellness with Wall Pilates. Far beyond ascetics or performance, true health syntheses physical prowess with mental clarity, emotional balance and spiritual purpose. The following chapters deliver all one needs to rebuild body and spirit for boundless personal fulfillment every year ahead.

Let your wall workspace guide inner reflection as you connect with core essence using my C.O.R.E. mindfulness method:

- Concentrate on proper breath and form in motion.

- Objectively observe all muscular and mental sensations without judgment.

- Respond slowly and patiently to body wisdom over ego demands.

- Empower self-care priorities daily, not just when strained or overwhelmed.

The C.O.R.E. approach ensures Wall Pilates serves you fully by reducing stressful mental clutter and reactive thinking habits. Mind-to-muscle flow motionAfter an exhausting day, Wall Pilates provides mental solace before physical strengthening. The wall cradles yet challenges body limits to channel stress productively. Discover renewed calm and confidence that ripples positively into all life arenas.

This book distills two decades of my award-winning Wall Pilates programming taught around the world from elite sporting camps to nursing homes. Core principles proven to realign every body safely by progressing foundational moves before diversifying intensity or equipment. Follow my blueprint to transform fitness, prevent pain, maximize mobility, and expand personal potentials daily. Continue honoring the visionary Joseph Pilates, who said it best regarding Contrology...

"You will feel better in 10 sessions, look better in 20 sessions, and have a completely new body in 30 sessions."

Let your Wall Pilates journey begin...

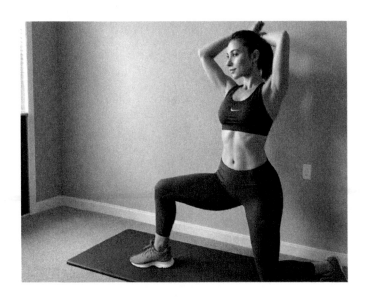

CHAPTER 1

GETTING STARTED WITH WALL PILATES

Welcome to the world of Wall Pilates! This powerful practice taps into Pilates principles of core strength and balance in unique vertical planes using just your own bodyweight. Get ready to realign posture, improve mobility, and transform fitness level safely with just basic wall space. Master fundamentals first before progressing to prevent injury and optimize results long-term. This chapter sets proper foundations before moving routines.

Assessing Current Fitness Level and Goals

First determine your current baseline fitness and limitations to customize Wall Pilates workouts effectively. Assess cardiovascular health, muscle tone/strength, weight, joint mobility and core stability honesty using the checklist below. Repeat assessments monthly to gauge progress. Compared to past peaks when younger or post-childbirth to set realistic targets relative to age, injuries and lifestyle changes. With accurate self evaluations, nurture strengths while addressing any weakness using Wall Pilates customizable programming. The wall adapts exercises to boost all skill sets gently.

Fitness Assessment Checklist:
- Cardiovascular Endurance - peak heart rate, VO2 max levels
- Muscular Strength/Endurance - reps based on body area
- Weight/Body Fat Percentage
- Balance/Stability - single leg stands duration
- Posture/Alignment - scoliosis, rounded shoulders
- Flexibility/ROMS - hypermobile, tightness areas

- Core Strength Test - front/side planks hold times
- Injuries/Discomforts - joints, disks, strains
- Energy Levels - stress, fatigue, burnout risk

With current fitness benchmarks established, reflect on lifestyle vision and purpose for your Wall Pilates practice. More than just aesthetic or performance goals, view Wall Pilates as a lifelong journey toward whole health - body, mind and soul. Consider both physical aims like muscle tone or weight loss along with mental/emotional aspirations like confidence, expanded potentials or self-love. Create an intention statement or mantra related to your highest wellness priorities then post visibly as daily motivation.

Here are sample fitness intention mantras:
- "I will be resilient to share my greatest gifts freely."

- "Balanced movement brings clarity of mind and openness of heart."

Revisit mantras often during Wall Pilates sessions - especially when frustrated or drained. The wall embraces during difficulty while keeping purpose aligned. By mindfully assessing fitness levels holistically, customize practices for safest fastest breakthroughs!

Safety First! Wall Pilates Guidelines

The wonderful thing about Pilates is adaptability across all levels from elite athletes to seniors. Listen to your body always and pull back or stop if pain emerges. Build gradually instead of rushing advanced moves before establishing solid foundations first. Master technique before intensity for longevity free of chronic strains. Progress comes pacing properly to prevent collisions between overzealous mindsets and exhausted capacities. Grow patience as

Pilates repatterns years of postural or movement habits.

Here are key safety guidelines:

1. Breathe fully - don't hold breath that strains or tire muscles quicker. Inhale energizes, exhale facilitates deeper motion.

2. Pull shoulders down and back - keeps chest lifted for ideal alignment.

3. Draw navel inward to brace the deep core - protect lower back vulnerability.

4. Soften knees \ light grip of toes to stay springy.

5. Isolate specific muscle groups - no straining other areas.

6. Micro-movements are effective when done precisely over speed or range.

7. Hydrate adequately pre/post session - muscles need water!

8. Warm up gently first especially if over 40.

9. Cool down slowly with stretches after.

10. Rest 1-2 days between strength sessions for recovery.

Pro Tip: If you feel strain in back, neck or hips during Wall Pilates stop immediately and regress range or intensity accordingly next attempt. Seek physical therapy guidance if sharp pains emerge.

Preparing Your Wall Pilates Exercise Area

One beauty of Wall Pilates relies on simply using convenient blank wall space available most places instead of bulky equipment or machines. Ensure the wall surface area selected allows you extend arms fully overhead without touching ceilings or move side to side unobstructed approximately 6-8 feet wide. Use sturdy home walls like living/bed rooms, durable building exteriors or outdoor structures weather permitting. Travel bands convert basic hotel rooms easily. Garage walls work great with yoga mats for padded ground support.

Ideally select wall regions with these qualities:

- Flat/Smooth Textured Surfaces - avoid bumpy bricks or heavily padded walls limiting grip/resistance.

- Dimmed Lighting - prevents glare eye strain. Overhead spotlights help observe form.

- Adequate Airflow - prevents overheating.

- Privacy from Interruptions - sets a safe mindset to move freely without self-consciousness.

- Upbeat Music - flows inspire yet not distract fully from body cues.

Experiment with walls in different locations for variety until discovering your ideal workout sanctum. Additionally consider setting your Wall Pilates zone during times feeling stressed for productive mental release or energized mornings for focused flow. Personally evenings recharge me best after sedentary workdays. Play with setup factors maximizing comfort, functionality and motivation for daily success!

Basic Wall Pilates Movements and Techniques

Now that your Wall Pilates area is set safely, explore fundamental footwork, arm positions, and practice essentials to ingrain properly before adding routines. Mastering these basics first prevents ineffective flailing or strain patterns. Quality trumps quantity always in Wall Pilates focusing on precision over pace. Envision moves unlocking from core center outward to limbs for injury free fluidity. We will break down basics in these key categories:

1. Foot Positions - ground control points
2. Arm Positions - counterbalance mobility
3. Core Foundations - center of all forms
4. Breath Basics - power / focus fuel
5. Rep Pacing - slow and controlled

Proper Foot Positions

Pilates foot positions differentiate from traditional upright exercise stances providing essential leverage, mobility and foundation. Note toe/heel relationships allowing springy moves in tandem with core and arms. Practice key options below:

- Parallel Feet - Toes/heels align facing forward. Distributes weight evenly through length of feet arches. Protects knees best for static moves like toe taps or small range knee lifts. Symmetrical parallel stance integrates the lower body evenly.

- V-Shape Feet - Heels together, toes facing outwards for thigh/glutes isolation targeting inner leg range. Feet also called first turned-out position. Protects knees while externally rotating hips for access. Common in thigh squeezes or standing adductor stretches.

- External Rotation - Rotating leg outward with foot arched initiates deep hip flexibility and thigh/glutes activation. Second turnout with heels separate wider amplifies internal thigh tension. Progress gradually while stabilizing the opposite leg. Targets hips, IT bands, inner thighs effectively.

- Tip Toes - Transferring weight forward to balanced toes boosted calf definition plus ankle stability and range. Ensure controlled form not straining arches excessively if issues present. Elevates heart rate for cardio bursts too. Excellent full foot mobility developer.

- Heel Lifts - Pressing just heels upward for micro rear glutes pump or during back extensions. Keeps quads relaxed for pure hamstrings/glutes isolation. Recommend holding the wall initially for balance assistance.

Now that essential foot positions are established, harmonize arms for optimal upper body toning and posture.

Ideal Arm Positions

Arms serve as counterbalance pulleys down the wall drawing out resistance while the core stabilizes. Smooth motions prevent shoulder overuse or neck injuries. Flow arms to facilitate - not force - range so other muscles progress gradually. Review options:

1. Shoulder Circles: Roll shoulders gently back then forward down for injury free joint mobility. Circles build rotator cuff strength while relaxing the upper body.

2. Front Raise: Lift arms actively from sides up towards ceiling without arching back. Palms can face each other, forward, or down which shifts shoulder muscles targeted. Upward scapula motion opens chests improving posture.

3. Lateral Raise: Arms rise away from sides of torso targeting middle deltoid heads. Avoid outward chicken winging by lifting shoulders down keeping elbows soft. Light weights increase lateral challenge. This move is found in all upper body dances.

4. Bicep Curls: Bending elbows pulling forearms towards biceps for peak contraction. Palms downwards activates the outer bicep most. Palms up shifts focus more on brachialis muscles nearer elbows. Vary angles for full upper arm balance.

5. Tricep Extensions: From bent elbows, straighten arms back feeling triceps pull down behind upper arms without locking joints. Counteracts bicep curls opening elbow joints fully.

6. Wrist Circles: Roll wrists gently with arms straight. Loosens forearms while mobilizing delicate joints preventing injury from repetitive motions during routines.

7. Hand Grips: Squeeze palms together while pressing arms away against resistance. Tensions arm webs while testing balance and shoulder stability. Engages many ignored upper muscles deeply.

Now integrate arm awareness into total body flows. Anchor shoulders down before piloting arms to challenging yet safe ranges.

Activating Core Essentials

The literal center of Pilates exercises boil down to core strength - abdominals, obliques, hips, pelvic and lower back zones that stabilize moves then transfer power outward to mobilize limbs. Core also centers breathing patterns before fueling blood flow. Master basic activation below:

1. Neutral Spine: Stand with back cradled against wall arms at sides, elbows soft. Feel the entire spine length, pressing gently back from tailbone to neck without collapsing chest forward or overly arching low back.

2. Shoulder Blades Down/Back: Draw shoulders blades down toward hips then rotate blades rearwards. Opens chests for proper lung inflation while preventing rounded slouching.

3. Pelvic Tilts: Tip pelvis forward then reverse to tilt rearwards without collapsing posture. Develops lower core awareness essential for hip/low back safety.

4. Navel Draw Inwards: Actively pull navel area up under rib cage without fully holding breath. Creates corset-like support protecting spine similar to natural brace before contact. Forgotten by many!

5. Peripheral Muscles Tension: Gently squeeze muscles at the total body periphery from thighs, glutes, forearms and even faces! Creates stability foundations before motions begin.

Practice the above steps sequentially until each one flows naturally as a daily posture habit. Walk taller with navel lifted and shoulders anchored to decrease back strain plus open lungs fuller. Next layer basic breathwork.

Breath Basics

Far beyond oxygen intake for muscles, Pilates breathing synchronizes motions with power generation from expanding lung pressure while exhales facilitate deeper movement. Inhale typically energizes lifting postures while exhales assist increased mobility or range like an accordion pumping. Practice breathing foundations:

1. Box Breathing: Inhale fully visualizing air filling torso up, front and sides then exhale pressing lightly inwards all around. Use for warm up or rest cycles between exercises.

2. 2:1 Breath Ratios: Move for 2 counts on inhale pauses then extend further or open during 1 count fuller exhale. This eccentric patterning protects joints while enhancing range of motion.

3. Exhale Flushing: Adding breath release hisses while exhaling helps relax muscles further during mobility

stretches like cats/cows or quad pulls. Releases provide relief.

4. Alternate Nostril Breathing: Classic yoga technique places the pointer finger gently on one nostril while inhaling deeply through the opposite side nose then switches the repeating pattern. Calms the nervous system, reduces anxiety levels and sharpens mental focus beautifully.

Proper pacing now builds a longevity base preventing chronic injuries down the road!

Repetition Pacing Perfection
Do not rush sets but rather embrace each concentrically through both physical and mental awareness for compound revitalization. Target 8-15 reps ideally with micro pauses between. Place sticky notes on walls tracking weekly progress. Consistency compounds even through subtle daily

achievements. Let's examine rep range nuances:

- 1-5 reps - Pure strength and power without bulk for delicate or injury prone areas. Use light weights if any.

- 6-8 reps - Muscular hypertrophy for size and definition increases. Moderate weight challenges stability.

- 10-15 reps - Muscular endurance for stamina through sustained time under tension. Bodyweight base plus bands add intensity gradually.

- 15-25 reps - Cardio challenge burns calories quickly. Rhythmic fluid motions elevate heart rates exponentially even without weights! Works across high repetitions to demand constant tension through limited rest cycles. This strategy ignites metabolism in fat burning mode for hours after the workout concludes.

Wall Pilates integrates all rep ranges holistically depending on areas targeted and desired training response. Mix high/lower repetitions with micro progression for periodization leveling up without plateaus. Now let's seal this Pilates intro class with a centering exercise designed by Joseph Pilates himself!

The Hundreds Classic
This signature sequence integrates breath, arm/legs moves plus mental focus uniquely preparing the body and mind for any physical activity. Try it anytime feeling tense, tired or unfocused for quick renewal.

1. Lay on back arms long at sides palms down, press belly button toward spine and lock pelvis level.

2. Inhale through nose lifting arms a few inches actively off floor straight without tension (avoid shoulder crunching).

3. Exhale through pursed lips for 10 beats while simultaneously pumping arms up/down rapidly while keeping arms light. Legs can stay stationary or lift/lower for added challenge. That's 1 set.

4. Inhale again softly through the nose before repeating knee lifts with arm pumps again for 10. Complete total 10 cycles.

5. Focus on breathing pacing not speed. Work from the center with control, calm and quiet intensity within.

6. Slow arm/leg motions completely on the last set then lower back to the mat for integration.

Practice "The Hundreds" between Wall Pilates workouts to reinforce foundational form, breath capacity plus mental clarity. This routine never loses its' centering effects or ability to check physical/emotional state honestly. Next journey deeper into programming personalized Wall Pilates flows with Chapter 2 flexibility essentials before maximizing mobility. Keep surrounding the body with loving wisdom and patience as we grow together.

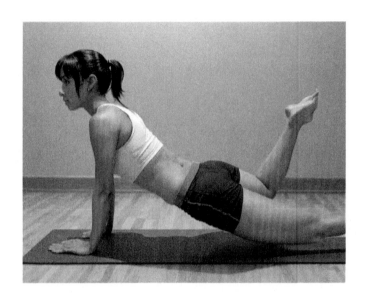

CHAPTER 2

WALL PILATES WARM-UPS AND STRETCHES

Just as construction crews require necessary inspections plus infrastructure reinforcement to uphold skyscrapers safely, our fitness foundations demand balanced flexibility to reach new heights. Warming up appropriately preps muscles, joints and connective tissues for increased demands during workouts while reducing injury risks exponentially. Stretches bring nutrients into constricted areas that boost functionality for daily wins. This chapter will guide loosening major muscle groups gently using wall support before diversifying movement ranges.

Warm Up Essentials

Think beyond cliché tropes of "no pain, no gain" that force progress ignoring body wisdom. Chronic issues and unwanted setbacks manifest from such short term quick fix mentalities. Respect innate edge levels to expand gently over weeks, not demand instantly daily. Create routines welcoming challenge levels appropriately over time through these safe warm up essentials:

1. Dynamic Motion First - Stationary stretching tight muscles increases vulnerability. Begin warming muscles in gradual sweeping motions using body weight shifting, light cardio elevation and mobilizing joints slowly through partial range of motion first. This increases blood and oxygen circulation to muscles, enhancing tissue elasticity.

2. Foam Roll Tight Areas - Applying gentle pressure against muscles and connective tissue with bodyweight melts away adhesion or scar tissue from strain or injuries. Feel for denser tight zones and breathe into pressure, holding tender points for release. Slowly add pressure as comfort allows.

3. Micro-Movements - Decompress joints with small rotations before widening circles to end range mobilization. For example: ankle rolls then toe/heel taps, neck half rotations becoming full head rolls, pelvic tilts adding gentle sways. Lull joints awake.

4. Breath Inspired Stretching - Extend mobility or flexibility range only possible through steady nasal inhale breaths fully then control ranges on complete exhales. Breathe into each

new edge before advancing further. Exhales relax and open spaces deeper.

Perfect progressed warm ups require equal parts patience and body awareness. Next practice stretches using wall support for deep tension relief across every major muscle group.

Upper Body Wall Stretches

The following wall assisted upper body warm ups boost circulation into tight chest, shoulders, biceps, triceps, forearms and wrist zones. Master opening this region before strengthening avoids overuse strains later from muscular imbalances or poor biomechanics.

1. Chest/Shoulder: Place forearms flat on the wall at shoulder height, step back until tension emerges. Breathe while allowing upper back to round freely for full pec minor/lat relief. Hold 2 minutes,

rock side to side gently over tender areas or modify arm height accordingly.

2. Lat Stretch Clasp: Set feet halfway from wall, extend arm straight up , pull to opposite side bent behind head. Clasp bent wrist with opposing arm then sit into hip gently until shoulder tension subsides while stabilizing torso upright. Switch arms while breathing fully for 2 minutes beside the wall. Enhances spinal rotation depth.

3. Triceps Stretch: Position one arm up overhead with palm flat/fingers forward. Grab the elbow of the same arm with the opposite hand then gently pulse the arm across the midline of the head stretching the triceps sweetly. Remember light neck support with a free hand. Hold tender areas then repeat the other side.

4. Wrist Flexor Relief: Start with the forearm along the wall then extend the palm until fingertips rest on the surface, step forward until tension then hold. To amplify, gently cup your palm over fingers stretching your wrist further. Switch arms then interlace fingers pressing palms forward opening forearm muscles often inflamed from technology overuse and repetitive motions.

Target frequently used yet rarely strengthened muscles proactively protecting against inflammation or injuries down the road. Now dive into legs as athletes' power centers.

Lower Body Essentials

Our metabolic engines lose optimal functionality from hours of sitting, standing or highly repetitive sports moves. Ensure complete spectrum stretching using wall assistance for foundational lower body care through moves below:

1. Hip Flexor Release: Place one foot forward supported on wall with back knee resting on ground and torso upright leaning slightly forward until front hip tension surfaces. Support balance safely if needed until hips square centering. Hold stretch breathing deeply then repeat the other side - essential for countering tight hip flexors causing back strain and injuries with many athletes.

2. Hamstring Love: Lay perpendicular to wall hip distance away. Place one leg straight onto the wall while the other leg rests bent as base support. Fold at hip crease extending arms forward as able until hamstring sweet tension. Rest head down and breathe deeply

for recovery from daily walking strains. Number one cause of painful lower back and chronic knee issues emerges from tight inflamed hamstrings. Give them restorative elongation attention.

3. IT Band Relief: Cross leg resting on wall then hinge away from wall at hip lightly for increased rotational stretch capabilities hard to create standalone. Protect knees while fanning inner thighs open. Hip joints will feel incredible mobility freedom opening their full functional arcs gently this way.

4. Quad Pull: Facing away from the wall, bring one foot up stabilized with both hands above the knee gently applying pressure against the wall thus pulling thigh muscles greater than possible standing alone. Adjust foot height/knee angles for complete

proximal, middle and distal quad isolation. Remember to breathe fully on each side!

5. Gastrocnemius Stretch: Stand one foot forward leaning pelvis and chest toward wall arms extended straight. Step back foot stabilizing body as front knee maintains soft micro bent shape avoiding full hyperextension. Enable greater soleus and gastrocnemius tension relief from daily strains like running or jumping sports. Monitor stretch depths gradually.

Finish flexibility training on high note with a closing series designed by Joseph Pilates himself for complete body restoration leaving you energized for strength routines ahead!

Cat Cows Flow Finale

This yoga inspired full body sequence synchronizes breath and movement to decompress joints gently before closing stretches. Cat cows mobilize their spine in a sagittal plane while massaging organs and enhancing neuro-energetic balance beautifully.

1. Kneel on mat hip width hands below shoulders like cat pose.

2. Inhale drop belly lift chest look upwards into cow arch.

3. Exhale pull abs up round back tuck chin towards chest for cat pose.

4. Move continuously for 90 seconds then hold the final cat pose pulling knees hips distance apart for deep hip opener sequence.

5. Walk hands forward into downward dog pulling its bones up and back.

Pedal heels bent knees easing lower spine.

6. Roll gently standing stacking spine bringing arms last overhead. Finish any tight areas with supported wall stretches before concluding rituals.

Fluid flexibility originates from balanced strength we will build together through programming progressions ahead. But first reward the body for all personal breakthroughs thus far with the deepest heart filled exhale yet! Your inner power, motivation and capacities to heal infinitely expand from here forward. Keep nurturing self lovingly as we flow...

The Power of Flexibility

Beyond physical gains, opening the body sensitively unlocks vitality and inner confidence too often dormant within routines. Tension builds mental rigidity and reactive thinking over time which spills into body armoring. Softening around areas of chronic tightness facilitates new levels of self-acceptance. Compassion towards limitations cultivates patience giving goals space to manifest optimally. Flexibility fine tunes awareness of neglected signals and instincts essential for navigating life's unexpected twists. What initially releases muscular knots transforms into renewed trust in innate abilities to handle uncertainty strong and centered.

Make decompression as much priority as strength progressions. Allow time rebalancing areas once deemed liabilities into liberating assets again. Whether previous injuries, illness or emotional trauma, blankets of protection cut off connections to whole self-worth. Peel restrictive layers gently with self-love, grace around setbacks and faith in inner healing wisdom. Support your body lovingly as we rebuild together.

See each Wall Pilates warm up and stretch as journey inward more than linear drive towards outward ideals. True power aligns inner beauty with outer physique through compassionate consistency, courage despite fears of inadequacy and celebrations of incremental self-expansion. The wall reminds us greatness comes slowly, layering small steps steadfastly. What flexible foundations allow is exponential growth when aligned to higher purpose. Allow your Core Essence first to guide outer transformations ahead.

Quick review of what you gained from our flexibility training:

- Dynamic mobility prep before stationary stretching
- Identifying and releasing muscle/fascia tightness
- Joint decompression and nurturing soft tissue

- Using breath work to enable safe range of motion
- Balanced strength and flexibility for optimal function
- Mindset shifts from rigid perfectionism to self-acceptance

This comprehensive warm up guide prepares muscle groups optimally for the strength, power and cardio challenges in coming chapters. But first reward the body with rest and high vibe nutrition fueling next level performance. Return only when fully integrated for peak energy, safety and focus. Avoid bulldozing fatigued muscles which leads to repetitive strain or acute injuries requiring even lengthier recovery downgrades. Consistency compounds long term just as flexibility followed by strength equals expanded potential.

Onward we rise together!

CHAPTER 3

UPPER BODY AND ARM STRENGTHENING

Let's build upper body strength, tone muscles and support healthy shoulders/wrists safely. This chapter guides you through leveled arm, chest, back and shoulder exercises using wall support for stellar posture and injury prevention. Master beginner movements before progressing variations to avoid overexertion. Review common mistakes to refine form optimizing results. Integrate gentle joint mobility warm ups we learned prior. Balance pushing and pulling moves for symmetry across muscle groups. Upper bodies thrive through a blend of tension, traction and mind-body finesse. Let's raise fitness peaks to new heights!

Activating Arms and Shoulders

The upper limbs connect core power to the world dynamically while also revealing posture imbalances quickly if shoulders rounded forward or wrists lack support. Pull shoulders back and down before initiating arm sequences. Soften elbows and relax neck to maximize results without strain. Target common areas prone to tech overuse or weakened through lifestyle habits:

➤ Shoulders - stabilize mobility plus transfer power from core rotational torque

➤ Biceps - pull weight towards shoulders for peak contractions and arm curves desired

➤ Triceps - straighten elbows with power after bicep curls to fully extend ranges

➢ Forearms - rotate wrists and grip objects with strength despite small muscle size

➢ Deltoids - round caps covering shoulder joints providing attractive shape and joint integrity

➢ Trapezius - triangular upper back muscle raising shoulders up/in as well as down/back together

➢ Latissimus Dorsi - broadest back muscles running along spine like angel wings for posture support

Let's begin with bicep build up before hitting surrounding groups!

Bicep Burners

Stand facing wall with feet hip width apart holding onto wall edges shoulder height. Protect elbow joints by keeping them midrange - not fully extended or bent. Avoid arm chicken wings flaring out by drawing shoulders down firm throughout motions.

1. Bicep Curls - With palms facing up, bend elbows pulling hands to shoulders feeling bicep bulge. Control returns without slamming joints. Add micro pulses once fatigued for deep burns!

2. Zottman Curls - Begin regular bicep curls then rotate wrists once contracted switching to palms down while slowly straightening arms. Twice the tension for fast firms!

3. Wide Grip Curls - Place hands wider than shoulders on wall edges challenging arms at distinct angles compared to traditional curls. Vary hand positions often.

4. Resistance Band Curls - Add levels by wrapping stretch bands around wrists pulling outward against eccentric bicep squeezes. Band pull forces harder contractions shortening muscle faster. Bands travel easily intensifying basics endlessly.

Triceps Toning

Press palms flat on wall shoulder width and at eye level. Set feet halfway between wall and parallel body, hips pulled back. Avoid leaning weight on hands by engaging the core fully. Protect elbow joints with soft micro bends.

1. Triceps Dips - Bend elbows lowering body gently towards wall then press up powerfully feeling triceps straighten arms fully. Add pulses once burned out.

2. Overhead Extensions - Step one foot forward as base. Raise one arm up, placing palm on wall while opposite hand holds elbow. Press arm overhead stretching tricep sweetly. Switch sides.

3. Diamond Push Ups - Bring palms together forming diamond shape. Bend elbows lowering chest towards hands on wall then power up keeping back straight. Intensifies tricep demands using bodyweight.

4. Kickbacks - Stand sideways with one arm up supporting upper body weight while the opposite arm stays parallel. Bend working arm then kick straight back only moving forearm and squeezing triceps. Protect elbows by avoiding locking. Challenging balance focus too!

Now integrate opposing pull moves hitting surrounding muscles often underworked.

Rear Delts and Upper Back

Pull muscles balance rounded shoulders for injury resilience through daily tasks like driving, typing or holding babies/pets. Squeeze shoulder blades together opening chests for whole body realignment benefits.

1. Bent Arm Angels - Raise arms to sides shoulder height keeping soft elbow bends. Slowly pull elbows back together like wings while widening against the resistance band above head fully opening chests. Lower with control.

2. Reverse Flys - Place forearms on the wall at chest height. Retract shoulder blades squeezing together to lift arms straight from the back feeling upper fly

muscles contract. Lower then repeat with controlled form.

3. Band Pull Aparts - Loop stretch band at chest level and press straight arms out against tension pulling band ends rearwards. Draw shoulders down and back. Constant time under tension repetitions boosts definition.

4. Wall Crawls - Place palms wide on wall walk fingers incrementally upwards while resisting gravity. Move your hands at snail pace to increase upper back tension beautifully. Intensify by walking fingertips backwards down using core control.

We have unlocked arms and upper back but don't forget mid and lower traps through integrated sequences next.

Rotational Strength Training

The largest yet most neglected muscles ride along spine length connecting shoulders to hips for protecting this vulnerability. Traps and lats stabilize upper movements yet commonly tighten from daily strain leading to headaches or injuries. Release then integrate routine based moves.

1. Wall Angels - Standsupported feet forward, sweep arms up overhead into gentle back arch feeling entire spine decompress then press palms on wall rolling down slowly through each vertebrae stacking until base. Mobilize in both directions with focused breathing for postural mobility.

2. Wood Chops - Stand side lunged one foot forward, hand high on wall. Reach up and powerfully pull diagonally down across the body like swinging an ax for integrated core rotational strength. Lead from the center then

switch sides. Chops also elevate heart rates!

3. Twisted Crunch - Lay body in plank against wall cradling elbows bent while rotating hips/legs openStack knees sideways then lift top leg to ceiling isometrically without hip drops engaging obliques fully before lowering with control. Master isolation.

4. Band Oblique Taps - Anchor band horizontally then tap front foot slightly out wide then cross over body behind working internal/external obliques in continuum. Mix speeds/heights for multi plane focus.

Finish upper body with our signature wall push up flows fully integrating arms, shoulders, chest and backs for chiseled 360 degrees gains sculpting power centers.

Wall Push Up Flows

This ultimate upper body toner sculpts every angle from delta to triceps using scaled versions of traditional push ups. Modify hand positions to shift tension across pectorals, biceps and axial core for6 pack benefits too. Bend elbows pulling chest forward then push back powerfully. Add micro pulses once exhausted by small fast bounces usingPartial range of motion. Flow through levels using box breathing inhales during lowerPhase and complete exhales while squeezing upwards. Let's elevate!

1. Wide Grip Push Ups - Set hands outside shoulders or halfway up wall if less stable opening chests further demanding greater strength stabilizing shoulders compared to narrow versions.

2. Close Grip Push Ups - Place hands at lower wall edges underneath

shoulders for more triceps demands keeping elbows tucked inwards to sides. Intensifies upper arms quickly.

3. Staggered Grip Push Ups - Set one hand elevated from the other alternating heights each set to require whole body torsion strength emphasizing core rotational stability.

4. Decline Push Ups - Elevate feet on chair slowly increasing incline angle to shift resistance burden from upper arms down to lower pectorals below chest muscles. Handles strengthen too!

5. Diamond Push Ups - Shift hands entering into diamond shape with pointer fingers and thumbs touching to isolate triceps for sculpted horseshoe detail. Intensify using hand spacers if available.

6. Fingertip Push Ups - Elevate wrists placing just finger pads on the wall demanding extra grip, forearm and bicep tension for auxiliary shaping.

7. Bokken Push Ups - Stack hands atop one another as if holding a sword to carve out inner chest lines with greater shoulder tension on stabilization. Samurai approved!

Finish floor routine with 90 degree arm holds challenging muscles to fight gravity before releasing pump by straightening elbows fully with control. Increase holds weekly until able to hold for 60 seconds. Remember to breathe fully and embrace sweet shakes as a sign of expansion ahead. Now reward the upper body with nourishing proteins for rebuilding plus calming stretch as we restore together. Onward and upward!

CHAPTER 4

CORE AND ABS CONDITIONING

Welcome to your core strength summit! This full spectrum chapter guides activating often dormant muscles spanning from pelvis, hips, transverse abdominals, obliques, serratus and lower/mid back zones. Review anatomy first before isolating muscle groups through leveled wall flows. Progress foundation moves before attempting advanced variations. Master precision alignment over pace. CoreTap inner power ready for new peaks in performance, posture and protection from daily strain. Let's start from the ground up!

Core Anatomy Essentials

Far beyond six pack abs, the true core comprises over 30 muscles that stabilize, mobilize and strengthen bodies dynamically. Review basic anatomy and roles below:

Pelvic Floor and Hip Muscles

- Located at base connecting upper and lower halves for fluid movement transfers when walking to jumping. Hug inward and upward towards the belly button.

Transversus Abdominis

- Innermost abdominal layer running horizontally like a natural girdle for heavy lifting support and slimming waistlines. Actively contract before any major motions.

Rectus Abdominis

- Outermost vertical abdominal muscle cuts between ribs down towards pelvis known as six or 8 pack shaping when developed. Flexes spine for curled positions.

External and Internal Obliques

- Crisscross muscles on side waist areas that facilitate multi planar rotations like golf swings across the body and protects organs laterally. Very important yet often the weakest link. Let's prioritize their toning together.

Quadratus Lumborum
- Lower back muscles beside the spine that facilitate transnational movements like side bends while preventing strain. Can inhibit side waist slimming if over tight. Stretch them daily.

Erector Spinae
- Muscles spanning full spine length wise from neck through low back that stabilize torso for standing, lifting and vertebrae protection. Prone to tightness from seated strain.

Master basic anatomy first before optimizing core conditioning connections for stable, strong centers ready for any activity!

Core Essentials Programming

Now integrate movements targeting each area through progressive wall flows to hit upper and lower zones. Master beginner moves before advancing for safety. Focus on precision breathing over pace or range depth. Create full spectrum core stability with balanced strength training.

1. Dead Bugs: Lay on back resting shoulders as base. Alternate lifting opposite arm overhead while lowering opposite leg straight for deep connections linking shoulder to hip mobility across torso. Advances coordination essential for agility.

2. Wall Planks - Place forearms flat on a wall leaning body gently forward

activating full front core and hips without straining lower back or wrist joints. Start conservative with angle and time then progress weekly. Most fundamental yet dynamic move strengthening over 30 muscles at once!

3. Wall Squats - Stand against wall then slowly slide down bending knees hips distance apart until creating 90 degree seated position against wall monitoring lower back arching. Build gradually thigh and glute strength able to support heavier weights later for leg presses.

4. Wall Sits - Place yoga block supporting mid back scooped forward to flatten spine against surface. Walk feet out while pressing both quads and calves parallel strengthening legs through sustained isometric time under

tension. Simply remove the block once stabilized for free standing variation.

Take core basics into daily life with improved natural mobility, balance and protection against strain or sudden falls. Now progress core challenges using the physics of wall spaces.

Dynamic Core Progressions

Take Pilates principles aerial through smart wall spring leverage for suspended core activation challenging stability unlike floor moves allow. Conquer the following lifts, lowers and holds first before attempting advance exercise variations. Master form before adding speed or weights.

1. Straight Leg Lifts - Lay body sideways, extend legs straight at hip level hinging from low spine keeping core lifted. Raise top leg upwards with control emphasizing lifted hips the

entire range of motion. Lower without arching back using core strength not straining neck or shoulders.

2. Knee Drops - Face wall slightly angled with soft micro bent knee held lofted while anchored standing leg sustains upright posture security. Release lifted knee gently down continuing support from base protecting knees and hips. Control feels more effective than range here. Lift knee back to start position with precision.

3. Bottoms Up Press - Lay below wall bridge style with arms extended straight holding light ankle weights (2-5 lbs). Maintain neutral press spine lengthening tailbone towards heels while lifting hips skyward emphasizing core muscles over straining neck. Use breath power inhaling up, exhaling lowering without arching low back at

floor. Option to pulse once inverted for deep burn and shoulder stability enhancements.

4. Plank Circles - Maintain straight plank position arms under shoulders while slowly tracing clockwise waist circles fully engaging obliques dynamically before reversing directions likewise. Intensify by elevating the opposite leg straight maintaining steady breath and posture throughout. Challenging rotational strength developer!

Now maximize powerhouse with isolation techniques for 6 packs and slender obliques beloved in swimsuits!

Rippling Abs - Oblique Slimming

The ultimate Pilates prescription reveals lean physiques through accentuating natural waistlines, carving ab definition plus trimming love handles simultaneously. Use wall traction resistance applied properly to expedite upper and lower rectus sculpting hiding below protective fat layers (no crunching required!). Strategy here relies on sustained muscular time under isometric tension. **Let's streamline slimmer together:**

1. Waist Slims - Stand angled sideways hips and heels pressed against the wall fully. Draw the belly button inwards then bend sideways creating intense oblique stretch upwards. Push ribcage upwards against resistance band wrapped above straightening waist creating micro lateral movements. Hold flexed waist pose squeezing obliques deeply before reversing stretch direction. Attain Jessica Alba level oblique curves!

2. Twisted Crunches - Lay body sideways wall plank style with elbows bent under shoulders, knees stacked on top

of each other with top foot lifted skyward working inner thighs and obliques simultaneously. Control drop top knee across body targeting deep oblique fibers while base elbow supports head neutral. Lift legs back to start position with perfect posture. Top leg lifts complement side plank flows for sexy leans!

3. Wall V-Ups - Secure body supine under wall bridge, arms long beside torso palms down pressing shoulders down. With straight legs trace giant V letter lifting hips skywards, legs overhead then open V sideways stretching inner thighs finally lower without fully resting feet down ready for next V-up repetition. Smooth transitions keep continuous tension for flattened stomachs quickly!

4. Lateral Leg Swings - Lay body sideways supported on forearm, knees bent stacked. Extend the top leg straight then powerfully swing it forward/upwards/backwards using hip swiveling momentum to sustain pendulum motions with core stability. Set reps then switch sides. Challenges balance with trimming results rivaling hours on elliptical. Yes to sculpted waistlines and strong flexible sides!

Now finalize fierce abs with Joseph Pilates signature hundreds series intensifying transverse navel fibers for fortified protective cores ready to empower personal goals ahead!

Joseph Pilates Hundreds

The classic 100s sequence synergizes breath, pumping limb movements and mental focus preparing the body and mind optimally for any activity. Perform anytime feeling low energy or after core training to fortify results.

1. Lay flat knees bent, imprint spine by pressing low back down. Contract lower abs drawing belly button towards spine.

2. Inhale peel head/shoulders off floor reaching arms forward.

3. Exhale curling up thicker through waist keeping chin tilted slightly down to prevent neck strain.

4. Pump arms open/close repeatedly like quick swimming motions.

5. Inhale for 5 pumps then exhale for 5 more without pausing for 100 total reps. Gaze towards the belly button to keep the neck relaxed.

6. Remain lifted holding stillness to feel abdominal burn upon 100 with control.

7. Lower down slowly vertebrae by vertebrae feeling back rib cage then head gently reconnect with floor keeping knees bent for integration.

Para los que hablan español En 100 en cien, mantén tu vientre apretado y enfoca tu mente. Hazlo diario y verás los resultados.

Regular hundred breaths build endurance strength across transverse and rectus abdominal zones like no amount of crunching ever can! By actively drawing the navel down towards the spine, external obliques and serratus muscles also maintain tension protecting organs, stabilizing torsos and streamlining love handles simultaneously. Practice daily even doing small sets incrementally. Combine along with side plank series earlier for best 360 abdominal activation and intercostals definition revealing chiseled physiques. But remember even six packs bloom from inner confidence, consistency compounding over quick fixes. Build mental muscle fortifying fitness intentions with consistent core strengthening ahead. Stay focused.

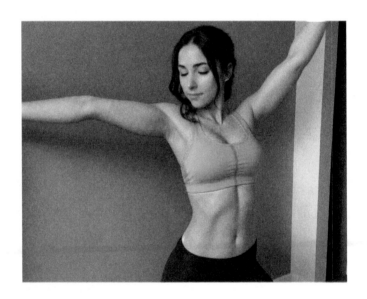

CHAPTER 5

STANDING LEG AND GLUTES WORKOUTS

It's time to tone legs fast and lift glutes higher using wall traction power facilitating amplified strength, shapelier contours and posture support like never before. Balance work builds lasting stamina while special footwork patterns reduce cellulite dimpling dramatically. We will integrate bands adding levels once basics are mastered first. Save intense routines for the cycle's end to allow tender muscles optimal rebuilding recovery between training avoiding strains or setbacks. Consistency sustains slow yet steady breakthroughs ahead. Let's sculpt famously strong toned dancer legs together!

Powering Up Posture Muscles

The core and legs share direct interconnected support. Tight hip flexors pull down abdominal walls and collapse posture negatively while weak inner thighs inhibit pelvic stability increasing lower back strain and compression. Rebalance this kinetic chain flow using moves strengthening from ground up:

1. Heel Raises - Stand with hands on wall lifting then lowering just heels concentrating contraction at the very top point of motion. Protect arches by avoiding slamming full feet flat down.

2. Toe Taps - Lift just balls of feet tapping gently toes and lowering control without unlocking knees sudden movements that jar joints long term Build intrinsic foot arches reducing pronation.

3. Plié Wall Squats - Set feet wide turned outward with heels planted, spine neutral. Inhale dropping just hips

directly down keeping chest lifted mimicking dance plié movement pattern. Straighten knees pushing evenly through full feet without locking back to start. Soften all joints.

Perfect plié squats targeting inner thighs and glute maximum muscle fibers building strong sturdy bases for increasing demands ahead. Let's dive deeper into weighted work now.

Single Leg Focus Flows

Split stance moves better isolate individual legs multiplying strength fast yet safely without straining knees or hips from heavier double leg versions initially. Challenge stability through planes of motion for functional durability:

1. Lateral Lunges - Stand sideways parallel to wall arms length away able to place one palm for support. Shift

70% weight slowly into one leg bending knee deeply over center ankle while straight leg stabilizes. Avoid knees collapsing inward by rooting from outer glutes and hip external rotators. Sweep sideways for 2 counts down, 1 count returning up to start position with control. Repeat 8-15 reps then switch legs.

2. Diagonal Lunges - Face corner angling body diagonally with hand touching wall overhead for balance.lunge one leg stepping wider not forwards working inner thigh while pressing from wall gently with opposite arm for core engagement too. Master form before adding dumbbells to challenge stabilizers greater.

3. Curtsy Lunge - Position legs staggered one forward, cross back leg behind front leg bending deeply into hips

really targeting external rotators. Rise up slowly with control. Intensify by holding dumbbells at chest heights like goblet squat. Hits oft neglected region!

4. Skater Lunge Jumps - From staggered legs, bend into lunge then powerfully jump switching front legs landing gently absorbing joints through athletic poses. Focus on hang time length challenges most advanced athletes!

Stand strong integrated now through unilateral stability boosts ready for glutes galore grabs ahead!

Lifting Glutes and Lower Body

Shape legs famously like dancers starting with isolated glute bridges before layering multi dimensional motions recruiting surrounding groups efficiently. Master moves below to lift legs into alluring contours quickly yet safely:

1. Fire Hydrant Kicks - Kneel on all fours, kick one bent leg out sideways leading with heel keeping hips steady and knee at 90 degree angle. Squeeze glutes at top of motion before smoothly returning knee down still bent protecting joints. Repeat 20 tiny presses then hold the leg lifted isometrically for deep burn!

2. Kneeling Leg Abduction - Kneel sideways parallel to wall for balance support. Keep body upright while lifting one straight leg directly out sideways working outer glutes and thigh sweeping moves before slowly lowering without twisting or dropping hips steady. Even micro movements effectively target tone trouble spots here keeping tension constant.

3. Frog Glute Bridges - Lay on ground knees bent feet wider than hips also turned outward for deep glute isolation. Press down strong through heels lifting hips high then lowering with control emphasizing glute squeeze each rep. Bands overhead or bars held increased challenges when mastered.

4. Banded Walking Glutes - Place mini loop band above knees then walk forward stopping each third step to perform mini squat working glutes through fullest ranges and surrounding groups by accelerating motions horizontally. Step and squeeze for rounded results!

Now put it all together for famously alluring lower bodies through our Pilates sculpting flow routine performed weekly!

Standing Thigh and Glutes Burner Flow

Let's sequence sculpting moves together for compounded lower body lifts through sustained sets. Perform circuit straight through without rest at steady tempo then repeat again 2-3x for transformation. Mix routines biweekly emphasizing heavy glutes focus one week then intensive thigh toner. Customize for addressing imbalances or personal shaping goals. Have fun watching legs upgrade radically through consistency looping these flows:

1. Sumo Squats
2. Side Lunges
3. Diagonal Lung
4. Fire Hydrants
5. Heel Raises
6. Curtsy Lunges
7. Frog Bridges
8. Toe Taps
9. Banded Walking Glutes

10. Wall Plié Squats

Repeat 3 Round Circuit 2-3 Times Through Weekly

Focus on perfect posture spine elongating up while sinking hips below parallel emphasizing plié technique fighting off knees collapsing inward. Move with steady tenacity through burning quads or early wobbling. Control motion smoothly resisting momentum for deepest gains. Pause only when form falters. Catch focused breath then continue full sets without distraction.

Upon final round completions, reward incredible efforts by relaxing fully onto back knees bent like goddess pose allowing breath massage worked regions deeply from within. Inhale visualizes healing oxygen circulating everywhere. Exhales release lactic acids, fatigue or doubts about capacities achieving goals. Each session strengthens physical and mental fortitude exponentially. Consistency cultivating over quick fixes grants the most radiant strictly muscular legs plus inner confidence to express your highest vision. We transmuted together thus now shine brighter!

Onward now we flow...

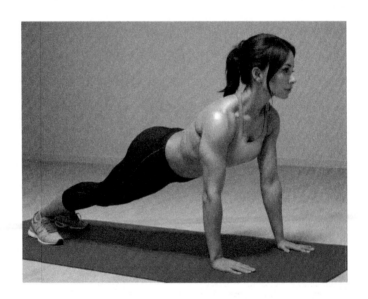

CHAPTER 6

SEATED LEG STRENGTHENING

Let's restore length and mobility across hamstrings, hip flexors, adductors, IT bands and quad muscles prone to daily strains from hours standing/sitting. Practice corrective stretches using walls for gentle traction before leveling up mat strengthening flows targeting athletic leg leanness and lift. Balance push/pull sequences to expedite muscle recovery, enhance facial sliding and maintain pain/injury resilience through demanding training phases ahead. Move slowly with precision feeling for trembling signals of true transformation. Let's begin supine integrating breath to unwind deeper now...

Restorative Hamstring and Hip Openers

The following movements counteract postural strains from frequent sitting, athletic overuse and even high stress levels manifesting physically as uncomfortably tight hips and legs. Use the wall securely to decompress identified problem zones optimally. Hold tender areas longer, breathing deeply into layers of tightness until sensation softens.

1. MyFigure 4 Glutes - Lay body perpendicular to wall and cross one ankle over opposite thigh into number 4 shape. Clasp hands behind bent knees then pull towards chest until sweet stretch emerges across glutes. Breathe fully into sensations for 90 seconds then switch crossed ankles repeating the opposing side. Excellent for opening external hip rotators and realigning sacrum.

2. Seated Forward Fold -Sit sideways legs extended resting against the wall. Inhale arms up then fold forward

walking hands out further feeling full back of leg lengthening. Pause pressure on any denser hamstring adhesions until breathing into them softens fibers. Round up vertebrae slowly with flat back to protect spine stacking properly. Decompresses lower back beautifully.

3. Half Frog Stretch - Begin seated straddling legs wider than hips pointing knees outward. Lean chest forward placing forearms on ground while flexing one knee upwards with foot inward pressing front thigh outward for deep progressive hip stretch. Gently sway hips side to side then forward and back releasing deeper still. Switch bent knee and repeat pushing opposing thigh outward into gentle rotations to coerce tingling!

Now integrate mat moves targeting quads, IT bands and adductors in continuum for supple lower bodies renewed.

Mat Based Leg Toners

The following Pilates sequences strengthen standing leg gains through equivalent seated resistance flows. Master first on carpet then progress to wall traction for increased load forces multiplying muscle gains faster. Emphasize control over depth or pace. Stop immediately if strain emerges. Breathe fully between fluid transitions. Let's begin supine warming up now...

1. Hundreds Legs - Activate powerhouse imprinting low spine down knees bent feet raised engaging quads isometrically Prepare arms halfway lifted then pump rapidly up/down while simultaneously extending one leg higher alternating sides keeping hips sturdy throughout 100 quick reps.

Hug navel deep into the spine the entire set. Burns legs exponentially!

2. Inner Thigh Squeezes - Lay on side supported on forearm place pillow between knees. Inhale adductors pulling knees together exhale resisting squeezing further. Quick pulses skyrocket heart rates while smoothing saddle bags. Stay lifted through the core for best results.

3. Heel Slides - On back gently slide one heel out along floor bending knee tracking over ankles then alternate sides controlled stretches decompressing quad muscles beautifully. Intensify gliding feet fully up the wall without arching low spine progressively. Increase range only as hamstrings relax deeper over time.

4. Bicycle Crunches - Interlace finger behind head imprint spine lifting shoulders while bringing one elbow towards opposite diagonal knee fully rotating torso targeting deep oblique fibers so important for strong legs and spines. Enhances proprioceptive coordination.

Let's diversify quad sculpting now upright against the wall integrating tubes for ratcheted intensity burnouts!

Against the Wall Athletic Leans
Stand with feet hip width leaning body fully back pressing spine against wall arms forward. This angled position allows gravity to assist quad engagement working legs deeply without compromising low back safety. Bands add levels for athletes while supporting balance. Let's proceed legs first before core flows:

1. Mini Squats - Bend knees lowering just a few inches working quads through fullest superficial ranges without straining knees. Concentrate on maximizing time under tension. Increase reps versus depth here.

2. Sumo Squats - Widen stance with feet turned outward sitting hips back and down keeping weight on heels. Pushes hips and inner thighs below parallel outside typical quad zone demands. Challenging!

3. Shoulder Press Side Steps - Hold light weights pressing arms straight up from shoulders while taking wider side steps working quads and hips stabilizers dynamically. Keep chest lifted throughout.

4. Lateral Walks With Band - Place resistance tube above knees taking

wider side steps forcing knees to stabilize against pulling outward demands firing hips and quads simultaneously.

Sneak peek into Chapter 7 flexibility reward waiting after today's deep burn finale quad toner together now!

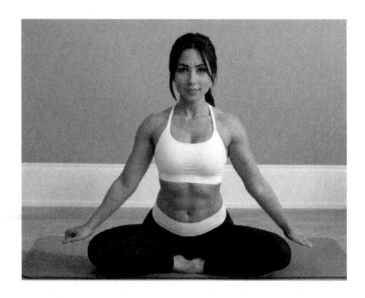

CHAPTER 7

COOL DOWNS AND FLEXIBILITY TRAINING

Total wellness extends far beyond physical gains or poundage lost on scales. Also prioritize nourishing inner resources otherwise every victory becomes sabotaged by debilitating levels of stress, fatigue or overexertion destroying even best laid health intentions overtime. Consider flexible lifestyle factors as important for progress as sculpting routines. This chapter shares Wall Pilates cool down essentials, whole body stretches, plus lifestyle changes supporting lasting success implementing new habits. Let's relax inside out now for peak performance training ahead.

Cool Down Imperatives

Far from time to zone out, cool downs seal progressive strength results optimally through specific sequencing and stretches to reduce strain, stiffness or next day aches retarding continued consistency. Follow these rules:

1. Attend any pain signals first stopping exertion then apply gentle compression to ease regions.

2. Initiate long deep breathing cycles to downshift nervous systems, let heart rates drop slowly and redirect blood back towards muscles. Oxygen fuels tissue rebuilding and metabolic waste removals best post workout.

3. Savor sweet endorphins and neurochemical side effects naturally uplifting mood and focus for hours afterwards. Smile wide, fully embracing internal highs from training.

4. Stretch in only pain-free ranges respecting tender regions, holding sweet tensions for anatomical realignments counteracting imbalances. Breathe into edges gradually, not forcefully.

5. Reward taxed muscles with overhead extensions, sways exaggerating spinal curves, gentle twists plus open seated poses that passively relax through gravity.

6. Softly massage neck, shoulders, wrists with soothing essential oils like lavender or chamomile. Let textures reconnect the sensory mind to present moment relief.

7. Consider alternating hot/cold water therapies dunking feet or hands that divert body mechanics deescalating

inflammation and reducing fatigue for faster turnaround next sets.

8. Refuel soon after with easy to digest proteins supporting muscle repair and naturally sweet anti-inflammatory foods promoting immunity, reducing cortisol and stabilizing hormones and metabolism affected by intense exertion. Eat clean. Hydrate 1 gallon water daily. Sleep deeper for 9 hours. Accelerate results integrating these lifestyle habits outside just training outputs.

Consistency relies just as much on strategic rest programming as correct strength progressions week to week. Now let's release full body holding patterns opening newfound freedom of movement ahead.

Wall Assisted Upper Body Stretch Flow

Target tightened areas prone from daily strains of driving, hunching over devices or holding tension across elevated shoulders, rounded spines and compressed torso zones. Open wrists, chests, hips and abdominals against wall traction for amplified range of motion rewards.

1. Wrist Flex - Straighten one arm fingertips pressing wall lightly, step forward until gentle wrist traction, hold 90 seconds gently cupping palm over fingers for deeper carpal tunnel relief if needed.

2. Lats and Chest - Place forearms stacked against wall straightening spine then sit hips back chest forward feeling sweet softening between shoulder blades. Allow your head to hang gently for upper back relief. Breathe fully.

3. Assisted Squat - Stand with heels touching wall feet hip width apart then bend knees lowering down wall into deep squat. Let gravity stretch hip flexors, quads and ankles dynamically over 60 seconds as tolerated. Option placing a yoga block or pillow under heels keeps toes engaged for stability.

4. Hamstring Stretch - Lie supine perpendicular to wall loop strap around arch of one foot straight leg onto wall hip distance apart. Micro bend working knee as flat leg lifts progressively up wall to sweet tension stopping prior overextending range to prevent cramping. Hold 2 mins each side.

Now cool tormenting cores, sides and hips with gentle assisted twists.

Seated Twist Series

Gentle twisting motions reverse compressive strains realigning spine and massaging away side waist tension. Use walls as leverage to control depths slowly. Allow breath guide range never straining. Deeper relief awaits around each corner...

1. Simple Twist Assist - Sit sideways extending legs front of torso bent knees stacked resting on wall. Walk top arm up behind you as the bottom arm presses gently against the front quad. Use core strength to resist collapsing as you eye gaze top shoulder further across midline. Swivel spine away from fixed hips. Hold then switch sides.

2. Half Lord of the Fish - From previous position straighten front leg placing same side ankle across body onto elevated knee quad hugging shin gently with arm. Gaze over the

opposite shoulder to guide deeper spinal rotations originating from the tailbone curling up each vertebrae sequentially. Squeeze glutes to anchor pelvis stable.

3. Revolved Crescent Lunge - Begin low crescent lunge with back knee down, ground front toes reaching arms straight overhead. Press bottom palm high on the wall , walk fingers down as you revolve your chest upwards through a tall spinal column. Circle arm across midline reaching long through energetic extension. Sink hips lower to feel juicy outer hip rotation stretch.

Finish with gentle symmetric cat cows waving spines supple inspiring renewed trust in body's inner wisdom ready for whatever lies ahead...

Cat Cows with Corkscrew Spinal Waves

1. Kneel on all fours imprinting spine neutral.

2. Inhale drop belly look upwards into cow backbend.

3. Exhale curl spine pulling belly up gaze to floor for cat arch.

4. Move continuously adding spinal waves flowing vertebrae by vertebrae in sequence.

5. Imagine center stripe corkscrewing alternating directions loosening the entire spine beautifully.

6. Allow the head to hang heavy, surrendering fully like wet noodles with each wave.

7. Close eyes turn inward, connecting breath to sensations swirling around the body.

8. Finish neutral spine relaxed child's pose for integration restoring length and space.

The Power Of Flexibility

Beyond physical tightness release, true transcendence unties mental and emotional restrictions accumulated over years reinforcing limited beliefs, rigid reactive thinking, pessimistic perspectives and doubtful worst case scenario attitudes. Gentle breathing focused stretching inadvertently softens armor protecting hearts from past pains or fears of future vulnerability. The Wall Pilates system thus intended transformations inside and out through compassionate self-acceptance, resilient progressions beyond perceived edge borders and embodiment of empowered potentials to serve the highest life purpose fully liberated. We nurture this uplifting community collectively through welcoming support, intuitive personal modifications honoring unique body variances and steady inspiration toward your highest wellbeing vision. Continue onward and upward leaning gently against Wall Pilates possibilities!

On behalf of the entire Wall Pilates family, thank you for the privilege of guiding your flexible foundations ahead. May inner peace and physical revitalization fill days with ease. Breathe fully. Smile wider. Shine on...

In closing, progress Wall Pilates moves through proper precision and pacing for individually appropriate results. Avoid comparison traps or timeline frustrations by keeping perspective centered on feel good mobility gains, not outcomes solely tied to scale weights or measuring tapes. What steadily builds over restless quick fixes grants for more meaningful rewards reinforcing positive fitness identities and lifestyle motivation compounding over years ahead. We cheer every little breakthrough together!

I sincerely hope you found this free sneak preview of the guide valuable with actionable tips improving your WALL PILATES programming and results.

You can purchase the full paperback edition of "Wall Pilates Workout For Beginners" on Amazon allowing quick access anytime to the proven fat burning and conditioning methods conveniently from your bookshelf.

While you're there, also check out my other top rated fitness books on strength training, bodyweight exercises and nutrition strategies taking your total health to the next level.

Author page

CONCLUSION

We've stretched through an incredible Wall Pilates journey together targeting all zones - upper body, core powerhouse, sculpted legs plus restorative flexibility finishes. Before we close, let's reinforce key programming principles for maintaining safe, effective home practices. Explore additional tips plus sample routines to customize satisfying your unique goals and ability levels. Lastly integrate lifestyle factors optimizing consistency, motivation and vitality taking wall workouts into the world dynamically. This flexible practice now fortifies daily life resilience beyond gym outcomes. Let's conclude strong together!

Additional Tips for an Effective Wall Pilates Practice

1. Warm up appropriately - Dynamic mobility before static stretching

protects muscles excitable to injuries when cold.

2. Hydrate adequately - Muscles require water and electrolytes to perform optimally. Dehydration deteriorates abilities.

3. Mindset mastery - Approach sessions using my C.O.R.E. method focusing inward through NON-judgmental Concentration, Objective Observations, Responsive pacing and Empowered self-care. Let go of negative self-talk or restrictive mindsets that sabotage fitness goals.

4. Emphasize precision alignment - Prevent injury by moving through a comfortable range of motions only without overexerting vulnerabilities. Quality trumps quantity especially for

beginners or when reconditioning post illness/injury.

5. Breathe fully - Maximize exercise efficiency by powering motions with strong steady inhales through nose, then exhale completely allowing greater mobility/flexibility. Never hold breath which strains muscles.

6. Mix up routines - Avoid plateaus by changing targeted muscle groups, adjusting challenge levels via speed/resistance or switching standing posture order. Add cross-training days too.

7. Counterbalance strength splits - Create programming hitting opposing groups on different days. Example: back/biceps together then chest/triceps. Reduces overuse injuries.

8. Address muscle imbalances - Don't ignore achy signals. Soothe regions asking for help then strategically strengthen lagging sides preventing chronic tears or impingements. Record daily metrics noticing trends.

9. Reward rest periods - Muscle groups require 48 hour rebuilding recovery minimum between intensive strength sessions. Schedule wisely and don't cram missed days. Consistency over daily grind mentality serves a greater long term.

10. Cue motions inwardly - Focus on working muscles intensely by mentally activating and squeezing areas through entire motions. Eliminate distractions pulling energy outward. Mind to muscle flow isolation shows fastest definition results.

Sample Wall Pilates Strength and Flexibility Routines

Use these professional templates below as guides scheduling personalized workouts specifically matching current ability levels, targeting unique problem areas and respecting time constraints realistically. Pencil in split routines gradually over week then tweak as needed. Consistency compounds fitness pays exponential dividends over years. Invest into your health wisely by committing just minutes daily. Let your wall anchor the first step forward!

Beginner Workout Split Option:
20-30 minutes 4x weekly

DAY 1: Total upper body + core Day 2: Lower body + Glutes
Day 3: Active stretch mobility Day 4: Rest/Cross-training

Intermediate Workout Split Option:

45-60 minutes 5x weekly

Day 1: Chest/Back/Core

Day 2: Legs Focus

Day 3: Cardio intervals

Day 4: Yoga Flow Flexibility

Day 5: Active Rest Stretch only

Advanced Workout Split Option:

60-90 minutes 6x weekly

Day 1: Push muscles - Chest/Shoulders/Triceps

Day 2: Pull muscles - Back/Biceps

Day 3: Leg Powerhouse - Glutes/Quad focus

Day 4: Core Powerhouse - Abs/Obliques

Day 5: HIIT Cardio Blast

Day 6: Restorative Yoga Flow

Customize your own utopian workout schedule reflecting current energy levels, time allowances and soreness feedback from muscle groups needing more rest days factored in. Review progress monthly massaging routines to prevent plateaus or overuse strain injuries. Our coaches happily help adapt exercises fitting unique cases like pregnancies, injury recoveries or illness setbacks requiring gradual re-conditioning management. Evaluate goals periodically and drop exercises proving too advanced or swap newer moves keeping curiosity peaked. Maybe add a warrior wall that runs outdoors for fun!

Motivation and Lifestyle Keys

Now extend fitness vibrancy into everyday lifestyle through these psychology boosts,self-care tools and nutrition bonuses amplifying wall workout consistency exponentially:

1. Inspiring Goal Visuals - Cut vision board images or quotes revitalizing personal drive during low motivation

moments. Watch who you follow online lifting spirits too.

2. Uplifting Music Playlists - Curate songs evoking happiest memories singing aloud triggering feel good biochemistry massaging the moment.

3. Accountability Partners - Invite mutually committed friends for extra nudge, keeping showing up through the temporary excuses phase. Celebrate little wins often!

4. Performance Tracking - Watch subtle improvements daily like added wrist push-up reps or hamstring stretch gains with flexibility. Small steps still count progress no matter the pace!

5. Mindfulness Stress Relief - If anxiety, insomnia or blues arise, tap back into the present moment using tactile

objects, listening to nature or quiet mediation noticing thoughts non-judgmentally without following reactionary emotions down drain holes. Keep perspective positive.

6. Schedule Self-Care First - Give wellness top priority status calendar blocking everything else around activity buffers. Less likely skipping sessions when planned ahead. Morning movement energizes productivity too!

7. Consistent Early Bedtimes - Muscles rebuild best getting 7-9 hours quality sleep in cool, calm environments. Maintain electronics curfew allowing deeper rem rejuvenation. Establish consistent rise/sleep cycles balancing hormones maximizing training performance.

8. Hydration Habits - Drink half your body weight in ounces of clean filtered water daily. Include mineral rich coconut water or fruit/herb infused options. Proper hydration enhances fitness exponentially.

9. Nutrition - Follow anti-inflammatory whole food diet emphasizing plants, lean proteins and healthy fats for nourishing muscle recovery, brain functionality and baseline energy upticks. Meal prep weekly.

10. Cue Gentleness - Glance in mirror replaced with appreciation for unique health journey over judgment. Celebrate feeling strongest ever today, not critique lagging parts still behind. Give thanks for the capability to move freely again! Our Wall Pilates instructors stand behind your goals committed through each little victory.

In closing this flexible fitness journey together, remember the most meaningful rewards manifest beyond just scale numbers, tape measurements or filtered selfies. What ultimately uplifts stems from inside out through courage, keeping commitments, self-love beyond appearances and trust in your inner wisdom navigating life's unexpected plot twists. Consider Wall Pilates more than momentary workouts but rather lifelong communities that compassionately build higher self confidence, embodied empowerment and deeper purpose connections benefitting all. We cheer every little breakthrough ahead!

Now shine brighter out there with centered strength and supple resilience gained from our Wall Pilates foundations built together. And remember true health means enjoying each breath fully while making the mundane magical again. Keep breathing deeply...

AUTHOR'S NOTE

Dear Reader,

I hope you have enjoyed exploring the world of Wall Pilates through the pages of this book! It has been an honor to share this unique, accessible, and effective approach to Pilates with you.

If you found value in this Wall Pilates beginner's guide, I kindly request just a few brief moments of your time to leave a review on Amazon. Your feedback will allow other fitness enthusiasts searching for at-home solutions to discover how Wall Pilates can benefit their strength, flexibility, and wellbeing journey.

Even just a line or two reflecting what you enjoyed or suggestions to improve future editions would profoundly support this book's reach so more people experience Wall Pilates wonderful whole body

revitalization. Plus your review motivates me endlessly to keep evolving Wall Pilates programming for all ages and abilities ahead.

I so appreciate you taking these transformative techniques off the page and into your daily wellness rituals. Here's to many healthy, happy years ahead thanks to the power of Wall Pilates!

With gratitude,
[RICHARD L. LYONS]